HGH Gel

The Safe and Practical Somatropin Human Growth Hormone

John P. Choisser

ISBN: 1724232959
ISBN-13: 978-1724232953

Note to readers If you are interested in purchasing or distributing Somaderm™, and have been referred to this book by an Independent Marketing Consultant, please be faithful to them and work through them. Otherwise, you may contact the author, who is also an IMC, through www.hghgelcream.com

New U Life's™ SOMADERM™ Gel is the only transdermal, FDA registered product containing homeopathic human growth hormone (HGH). Somaderm is perfect for the Low Dose, High Frequency dosage method that research studies have shown to be most effective. Efficacy statements have not been evaluated by the Food and Drug Administration. These products are not intended to diagnose, treat, cure, or prevent any disease. You should consult your doctor before beginning any homeopathic diet or nutrition regimen.

Published in the USA by Readerplace Books, LLC
www.readerplace.com

Dedication

To Coleen, for whom I hope to live a hundred and ten years. And for my daughter Cindy, who is a great proofreader.

Contents

List of Figures

Acknowledgements

I did considerable research before writing this book, and would like to acknowledge all of the researchers who have spent their careers learning and publishing their work on wellness and life extension. My hope is that their work will result in thousands of people living longer and more productive lives.

1. About this Book

Why do we need this book? There are several reasons: First, my scientific interest in health and nutrition has always made me curious about latest advances, and how they might be used to enhance our lives. Second, carefully-conducted and documented research into various forms of hormone replacement have produced very exciting results, and, third, the recent availability of a transdermal form of human growth hormone (HGH) now makes a low-dose, high-frequency protocol safe, easy, and affordable for nearly everyone. This book will explain why that is important.

Decades of research, including double-blind studies, have shown that hormone replacement using somatropin (the human growth hormone) therapy can offset many of the effects of aging. Furthermore, an outstanding feature of HGH replacement has shown that in small, natural doses, no side effects have been observed. And as we will see, low-dose high-frequency (LDHF) protocols have been shown to be particularly effective, mimicking the action of the natural secretion of the hormone in our younger years.

Another reason for this book is to offset some of the misinformation on the Internet about both the hormone and the various forms of therapy. One statement I noticed immediately on WebMD (of all places) was that anything that had an effect on nearly every body function was itself a reason for being skeptical. I would think that they would know that it is the *job* of HGH to effect every cell in the body, and therefore the function of that cell.

1

There are large books that go into great detail on these subjects, and I recommend them. This book is intended to present the results in a concise, understandable manner so you don't have to read all those heavy books unless you want to. But I strongly encourage any reader who wants to dig into the details (as I have) to get copies of these books listed in the footnotes, and to understand the excellent credentials of the doctors and scientists involved in the research.

Full disclosure department:

1. I am convinced that the availability of a homeopathic transdermal gel form of HGH is a very important anti-aging strategy that people should know about and use. Since using the product, I have personally experienced favorable changes in my sleep patterns and in my body shape. I am therefore an Independent Marketing Consultant for New U Life.™

2. Please read and understand the following: Statements in this book have not been evaluated by the Food and Drug Administration. These products are not intended to diagnose, treat, cure, or prevent any disease.

I would also like to repeat the request on this book's copyright page: If you are interested in purchasing or distributing Somaderm, and have been referred to this book by an Independent Marketing Consultant, please stay faithful to them and work through them. Otherwise, you may contact the author, who is also an IMC, through www.hghgelcream.com, or by email at johnchoisser@gmail.com.

2   About HGH

Our bodies are made up of a hundred billion cells, and they all act together to keep us functioning. What is it that coordinates this activity? The hormonal system is the communication system for dozens, probably hundreds, of body functions. And there are many different hormones, each with their own specialized function.

Consider the variety of cells involved: brain cells (neurons, for example), nerve cells, muscle cells, immune system cells, skin cells, digestive system cells, and on and on. Some cells are alerted immediately if you cut your finger, some are activated when you even think about food, and some rush to defend you against a bacterial attack. Some people think the immune system only goes to work when you get sick – but note that when you leave for the Happy Hunting Grounds you need to be refrigerated pretty quickly!

There are glands in your body that are in charge of producing and reacting to hormones. Some glands produce their hormones when they detect other hormones. Major organs, such as the liver, react to the presence of hormones to begin producing other hormones or substances to fulfil their particular responsibilities.

Source of HGH

In particular, the human growth hormone somatotropin (we will see the hormone has two names: somatotropin and somatropin) is produced by a tiny gland in the middle of the brain called the pituitary gland. In both men and women, its secretion normally occurs about three hours after a meal, after one hour of sleep, after physical exercise, and during fasting.

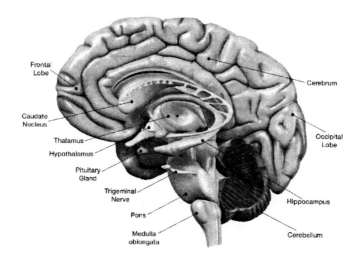

Figure 1.   The Human Brain, Showing Pituitary Location

HGH was discovered in the 1920's but was first used by Maurice Rabin at the New England Medical Center in Boston in the late 1950's. He injected it into a child with stunted growth whose own pituitary was unable to produce the hormone. The child's growth resumed to normalcy, and thereafter HGH replacement therapy became the standard treatment for these kinds of disorders.

The biggest problem initially was the scarcity of the hormone. It was being produced by the pharmaceutical companies by extraction from the brains from cadavers, which were in limited, and decreasing, supply. The supply was increased by the importation of human brains from Africa, but even then the problem of high cost remained.

Then the really bad news: some of the brains were contaminated with the virus that causes Creutzfeldt-Jacob disease, or mad cow disease as it is called in some places. It is a horrible disease, killing its patients in about five years after loss of muscle control and severe dementia. This caused the FDA to stop production and distribution of the hormone.

Several patients died, and those who had been treated with this contaminated somatotropin still might not develop symptoms for years after infection, making their lives miserable waiting and worrying.

Then the effort to synthesize the hormone began in earnest. A huge help was when congress passed the Orphan Drug Act in 1985, which rewarded companies that developed drugs that affected fewer than 200,000 people with exclusive production license for seven years.

Enter Herbert Boyer, a Nobel prize-winning scientist who founded Genentech in 1976. His company specialized in analyzing DNA, splicing it, and reproducing it by harnessing common bacteria to act as factories for these complicated molecules. For Genentech it was first insulin and then somatropin, the name for somatotropin made using recombinant DNA. Their somatropin worked, but was missing one amino acid (out of 191), but it didn't appear to affect its effectiveness.

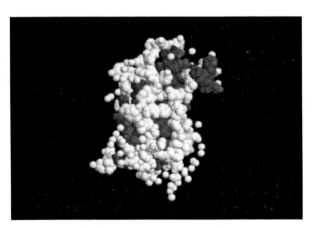

Figure 2.   The Growth Hormone Molecule Somatotropin

Eli Lilly improved on that by producing a growth hormone copy with all 191 amino acids shortly after that, and both companies began supplying the market with a pure, uncontaminated, and less expensive source. There are now about five reliable and high-quality sources for somatropin. Somatotropin from human brains is no longer used for safety reasons.

The Use Expands

In Madison, Wisconsin, an endocrinologist by the name of Daniel Rudman became curious about another important use of the growth hormone. He noticed that after the age of about 35 the human body begins to decline in step with the decline of HGH from the pituitary gland. Muscle mass decreases and the fat mass increases. The skin becomes thinner and wrinkled. The body as a whole becomes more defenseless against disease and injury. Mental acuity declines, and senility often ensues.

Moreover, in Sweden and Denmark, doctors who were treating stunted children had also begun treating adults whose HGH production was diminished by disease or other factors. They noticed that with HGH supplementation their adult patients were undergoing favorable changes in their body composition, such as increased muscle mass and decreased fat mass.

This made Rudman wonder if HGH replacement therapy could offset the "natural" decline in somatotropin production in aging (but otherwise healthy) adults.

Thus began studies too numerous to describe here, but available in the footnotes. To make a long story short, the studies, many double-blind, have all shown the effectiveness of HGH replacement therapy in offsetting many of the effects of aging. Some of the studies have helped refine proper dosage size and frequency, each study adding to the store of knowledge about the optimum use of somatropin.

As We Age

Many of the hormones produced by our bodies decrease as we age. A few don't, and actually a few increase. Unfortunately, HGH is one of those that decreases, along with estrogen (in women), testosterone (in men), and melatonin (in both). By the time we reach the age of 65, in most of us, HGH has decreased to less than 20% of what it was in our 30's. This decrease in natural somatropin is called the somatopause.

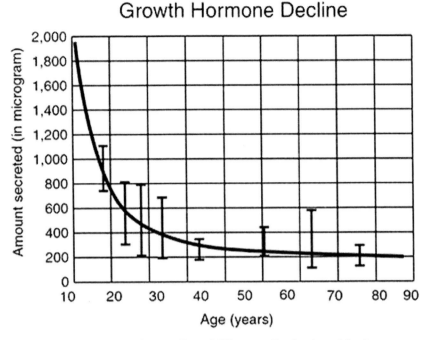

Growth Hormone Decline

Figure 3.   Decline in Growth Hormone Production with Age

Apparently, Rudman was correct. HGH replacement therapy can work to ameliorate many of the effects of aging. GHRP (growth hormone replacement therapy) has been the subject of many controlled studies, and they are yielding impressive results.

According to Ron Rothenberg, M.D., of the University of California, San Diego[1], *"We age because our hormones decline, not the other way around. GH is vital in order to live a healthy adult life. Why? GHRT improves quality of life. What other benefits does GHRT have? GHRT is beneficial to the brain, the cardiovascular system, the immune system, aerobic capacity, body composition, and bone."*

Not all endocrinologists are on board. As Dr. Rothenberg points out, *"they (some endocrinologists) are not in agreement with those doctors who believe in using GHRT to ameliorate the effects of aging. They agree that HGH supplementation is appropriate for children who don't produce their own hormone,*

[1] *Growth Hormone Replacement for Normal Aging*, Ron Rothenberg M.D., Clinical Professor/Course Director; Preventive & Family Medicine, University of California San Diego School of Medicine; Founder, California HealthSpan Institute, Encinitas, CA

and they agree that the same use is appropriate for adults with the same condition. They even agree that the benefits that are seen when GHRT is used on adults, they see the same improvements in the patients. But for some reason, they don't believe in using it on aging but otherwise healthy adults."

The symptoms of HGH deficiency in adults mimic accelerated aging. Research makes it very clear that the lack of HGH causes faster aging, and it is logical to conclude that as our own pituitary gland's output decreases over time, we continue to age. It is also logical to conclude that supplementing HGH as we age can slow the aging process, and such has been shown in many research studies by research hospitals, clinics, and universities all over the world.

3 The Effects of HGH Replacement Therapy

It should not be a surprise that because somatropin has an effect on every cell in the body, the benefits of its supplementation has wide-ranging benefits. This chapter will summarize the effects that have been observed by past typical (injection) studies.

How it Works

The hormone somatotropin is released by a normal pituitary gland in pulses, occurring a few times a day, depending upon your activities. The largest pulses occur during sleep, and smaller pulses occur after meals and exercise. It is interesting that pulses also increase during periods of fasting. Somatotropin only lasts minutes in your body, and works its magic by stimulating the liver to produce a substance called IGF-1 (also called somatomedin C). Because the IGF-1 is more stable and lasts longer in the body, measuring it is normally the method used in lab tests to estimate the amount of somatotropin being produced.

The following figure is from *Growth Hormone in Aging*, by Chertman, *et.al.*. It shows the somatotropin pulses over a 24 hour period. Note the small pulses after meals, and the larger pulses during sleep. Notice also the decline with age.[2]

---

[2] Lila S Chertman, MD, Mount Sinai Medical Center, Miami Beach, FL., George R Merriam, M.D., VA Puget Sound Health Care System and Professor of Medicine, University of Washington School of Medicine, Tacoma and Seattle, WA, Atil Y Kargi, M.D., Division of Endocrinology, University of Miami Miller School of Medicine, Miami,

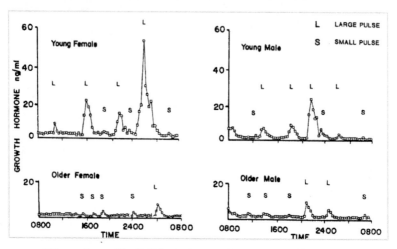

Figure 4.   Daily Variations in Somatotropin Production

The IGF-1 travels through the blood to every cell in the body, including those in the brain. Although HGH and IGF-1 are both large molecules, they both pass easily both ways through the blood-brain barrier. Because the levels of these chemicals decline as we age, down to less than 20% of that when we were 30, the objective of supplementation is to restore the levels of these substances to those previous levels. The remainder of this chapter will describe the observed effects that this therapy has had on research subjects.

Endocrine Web states that the generally-accepted effects of growth hormone *deficiency* on the body include the following.

- Anxiety and/or depression

- Baldness (in men)

- Decrease in sexual function and interest

- Decreased muscle mass and strength

- Difficult to concentration and lack of memory

- Dry, thin skin

- Elevated triglyceride levels

- Fatigue and/or tiredness

- Heart problems

- High levels of LDL (the "bad") cholesterol

- Insulin resistance

- Lower tolerance to exercise

- Reduced bone density, making you more susceptible to developing osteoporosis

- Sensitivity to heat and cold

- Very low energy levels

- Weight gain, especially around the waist

These effects clearly mimic those of aging. It should also be clear that, because HGH supplementation reverses those listed effects, that an opposite of the list would be the expected benefits of HGH supplementation.

Dr. L. Cass Terry, M.D., Ph.D., chairman and professor of neurology at the Medical College of Wisconsin in Milwaukee, analyzed 800 patients treated for two years between 1994 and 1996. He found that the levels of IGF-1 due to HGH supplementation rose from 238.8 ng/ml up to 384.5 ng/ml, an increase of 60%, bringing the concentration back to youthful levels.

Dr. Terry stated *"The most outstanding results were improvements in muscle strength, exercise endurance, and loss of body fat. Also, there were significant improvements in skin, healing capacity, sexual drive and performance, energy level, emotions/attitude, and memory. There were also significant drops in cholesterol and triglycerides. In general, these improvements occurred within 1 to 3 months and continued to increase over 6 months."*

Dr. Ahmad, of the Royal Liverpool University in England studied 22 women and 46 men who had pituitary glands removed for various reasons, thus resulting in Adult Growth Hormone Deficiency (AGHD). He concluded that *"Low-dose GHR (growth hormone replacement) improves body composition and QoL (quality of life) as early as 1 month after commencement and the beneficial effects continue at 3 months. Most importantly, these changes occur in the absence of side-effects. We therefore suggest the use of low-dose GH therapy, maintaining IGF-I between the median and upper end of the age-related reference range, for the treatment of AGHD."*[5]

There are literally hundreds of studies, many of which are described in Dr. Klatz's book on the subject. I highly recommend that those of you who want to dig into the details buy his books[4]. There are far too many success stories than can be quoted in this book.

Side Effects

The many research studies over the early years experimented with dosages, and all were done with the injectable form of HGH, which was all that was available.

General

Patients in studies that used large doses sometimes experienced minor joint pain and fluid retention that disappeared in the first month or two. Some studies using large doses showed some persistent side effects including carpal tunnel syndrome.

Modern studies are performed at doses much lower, and closer to the natural secretion levels the body expects from the pituitary gland, resulting in no reported side effects. Small frequent daily doses not only were shown as more effective than the larger doses, but showed no side effects. The most frequently cited risks for HGH replacement therapy involves cancer and diabetes.

Cancer

According to Dr. Klatz, it was most significant that there were no reported cases of cancer in the research subjects. Many researchers wondered if the growth effects of HGH would accelerate the growth of even previously undetected cancer, and people with cancer are still advised against HGH supplementation therapy.

However, that could be a mistake. Dr. Terry reported that *"With 800 people over the age of about 40 you would think that given the normal incidence rate of cancer, some of these people would get cancer. It could be that there is some sort of protective effect from growth hormone replacement."*

---

[3] Dr A. M. Ahmad, Research Fellow, Link 7-C, Department of Diabetes & Endocrinology, Royal Liverpool University Hospital, Prescot street, Liverpool, L7 8XP, UK.

[4] https://sile.amazon.com/s/ref=nb_sb_noss_2?url=search-alias%3Dstripbooks&field-keywords=Ronald+Klatz&rh=n%3A283155%2Ck%3ARonald+Klatz

Even more interesting, none of the male participants experienced an increase in PSA levels, and in one study, which Chien and Terry are going to report in a paper, a patient had a PSA level over 60, and a needle biopsy confirmed that he had adenocarcinoma of the prostate. Nevertheless, he insisted on participating in the study. After HGH supplementation therapy, his PSA declined to below seven. That may or may not constitute a cure, but it is an obvious improvement.

According to Child et.al., *"With relatively short follow-up, the overall primary cancer risk in 6,840 patients receiving GH as adults was not increased."*[5]

Insulin Resistance

New research is changing opinions on the effects of HGH replacement on the body's insulin resistance, and in the past, diabetics were warned not to use the treatment. Early in treatment, for the first month or two, the body's glucose tends to increase, which is a sign that it was countering the production of insulin, which is not a good sign.

However, Bengt-Åke Bengtsson, Medical Department, M. Aarhus Kommunehospital, Denmark, has reported that even though indications of insulin resistance appear in the first six weeks, after six months the indications were back to where they were before treatment began. He believes that the reason is that as the body's fat mass decreases, the body begins to normalize its reaction to insulin.

Clearly more research studies are needed, especially if it is discovered that HGH replacement therapy is good for diabetics rather than contraindicated.

Most physicians still do not consider aging a disease or disorder, and as we discuss the effects of HGH supplementation, we will also

[5] *Assessment of primary cancers in GH-treated adult hypopituitary patients: an analysis from the Hypopituitary Control and Complications Study,* Christopher J Child, Alan G Zimmermann, Whitney W Woodmansee, Daniel M Green, Jian J Li, Heike Jung Eva Marie Erfurth, Leslie L Robison, and on behalf of the HypoCCS International Advisory Board, 2011.

include some of the observed effects on disease other than aging.

Please note that all of the research reported in this section of the book are the results of studies using injectable somatropin, since the transdermal form has only been available for a few years. However, as you will see, the results so far appear to be the same.

HGH Effects on Aging

The effect of HGH on the liver and thereafter the rest of the cells of the body happens almost immediately, but change in some cells takes longer to notice than others. For example, we might be aware of brain cell changes in days, but skin, fat, and muscle cells might take months. The noticeable body change "schedule" that has been reported in research subjects is pretty well established, and will be described in more detail when we discuss what our expectations should be when we start low dose high frequency (LDHF) growth hormone supplementation.

The Brain

Even though the natural source of HGH is in the brain, until the past decade or so there were many researchers who erroneously thought that it had no effect on the brain. However, there are a growing number researchers that believe that HGH has much more effect on the brain than previously thought. In fact, many think that the common shrinking of the brain with age might be due to declining HGH production.

One reason for doubting the effect on the brain was the blood-brain barrier that normally keeps large molecules from passing through. (How they thought that somatotropin got out of the brain to the rest of the body without crossing the barrier escapes me.) HGH is a very large molecule, comprised of 191 amino acids. But when they injected subjects subcutaneously in the leg with somatropin, Dr. Bengtsson found that the amount in the cerebrospinal fluid increased ten-fold within minutes.

So what are the effects of HGH on the brain, and what results are observed? Below is a summary. If you dig into the literature available, you will see that each of the following paragraphs could easily contain many pages of case studies and reports.

Sense of Well-Being

One of the first reported results most people notice is a sense of well-being that is hard to describe. One person reported to me that it felt like some kind of relaxation behind her eyes. Another said that he felt like he could cope with life better. His job was the same, and so were his clients, his family, and his commute, but he didn't feel stressed out all the time.

It had been observed that children being raised in stressful, unhappy, and miserable conditions were not only unhappy, but also experienced stunted growth. This condition, known as psychosocial growth failure, responds favorably to HGH therapy even though there was no disease of the pituitary gland.

HGH injections have been shown to raise the level of B-endorphin while it lowered dopamine. This is the same reaction seen in patients treated with anti-depressants. B-endorphin has been nicknamed the brain's morphine, which, among other things, is the cause for the "high" many people experience after exercise (which increases HGH production in the brain).

Dr. Klatz reports that one woman testified that HGH replacement therapy was more effective in treating her husband's depression than Prozac had been.

Sleep

The second (or sometimes the first) reaction people report after beginning HGH replacement therapy is improved sleep.

Normally, the brain's secretion of HGH pulses are the strongest during deep sleep, and begin about an hour after going to sleep. Does the deep sleep cause the release of the hormone, or does the release of the hormone cause deep sleep? The answer seems to be the latter, since one of the nearly universal signs of aging is the lack of deep sleep. Poor sleep patterns increase as we age, which causes some to believe that older people don't need much sleep. But with good, deep sleep restored with HGH therapy, research subjects definitely don't complain about better sleep.

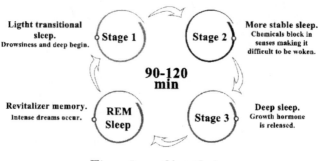

Figure 5.   Sleep Cycles

In fact, sleep deprivation results in decreased production of somatotropin, making for a miserable day after a sleepless night. Adults with severe HGH deficiency show very poor sleep patterns, with very short or few periods of low-wave deep sleep, and more periods of REM sleep.

Energy

In addition to the well-being feeling described previously, another side effect of HGH supplementation is increased energy. Perhaps this is due partly to improved sleep, which would not be surprising. But Dr. Bengt-Ake Bengtsson, a Swedish pioneer in endocrinology, noticed that fatigue was a common symptom among his HGH deficient patients. Growth hormone replacement resulted in "a great wake-up call" restoring vitality and energy to these patients. Researchers at St. Thomas in London also reported a great increase in their patients' energy and sense of well-being.

Growth hormone very quickly has an effect on body water. Part of the observed effects on energy and vitality might be due to the fact that cells respond to hydration by increasing their metabolism. Body cells lack of sufficient water shows up in shriveling skin and sluggish behavior. The opposite of youth!

Vision

I'm sure most people would agree that one of the first signs of aging is a decline in their vision. Even before gray hair or pot bellies, many people start buying reading glasses.

As we age, the lens in the eye loses elasticity. That keeps the lens from achieving the fatter shape necessary for near vision. In addition, distance vision also degrades, along with the eye's ability to adapt to brightness changes.

After a month or two of HGH supplementation, many patients have reported improved vision in some surprising ways.

- Improved near vision

- Faster adaptation to brightness changes

- Improved night vision

- Perception of brighter colors

There have also been many cases of help in diseases of the eye. One patient, reported by Dr. Klatz, had consulted several ophthalmologists regarding his macular degeneration, and concluded that nothing could be done. One of the doctors, however, recommended that he try HGH supplementation, and he began to experience improvements in his condition. His vision improved from 20/200 to 20/40 over a period of two months.

Memory, Cognition, and Reflexes

Patients on HGH replacement therapy have seen dramatic improvements in all three of these areas. Dr. Klatz reports one patient whose memory had deteriorated to the point that he would put a sticky note on his dashboard to remind him of where he was going. That's a little worse off than most of us, but as we age nearly all of us find ourselves going into a room and forgetting why. Or having trouble coming up with someone's name. Or losing the car keys.

These things are not necessarily a sign of disease, unless you believe, like many doctors now do, that aging is a disease. Jan Diejen and his team of scientists at the Free University of Amsterdam studied many of their male patients who either had defective production of pituitary hormones, including HGH, or just HGH alone. They found that the deficiency of HGH resulted in poor short term memory, long term memory, and hand-eye coordination. They also found that HGH-deficient people, particularly those deficient since childhood, had lower IQ's and had not progressed far in education.

Can HGH replacement therapy improve these conditions? According to Dr. Klatz, the answer is yes. Patients on HGH supplementation report improved memory, increased alertness, and faster reflexes. There are tests that can measure these things, particularly the game Concentration, the skin pinch test, and the reflex test using a falling ruler. More about those later.

There is evidence that boosting HGH can rejuvenate, repair, and stimulate cell growth in the brain, adding evidence that it is the lack of HGH as we age that causes the brain to shrink, not the other way around.

The author encourages the reader to study some of the references in this book, particularly Dr. Klatz's books, because there is far too much research going on to cite here. Supplementing HGH is showing very exciting promise even in treating brain diseases like Parkinson's and Alzheimer's. This is also true for the possible treatment for certain brain injuries, including stroke.

Of course research into the literature will also disclose opinions that differ from some of those cited in this book. That should be expected, since historically there have been very few advances in science that have received instant acceptance. Most of the controversy, however, seems centered not on the benefits of low-dose high-frequency HGH supplementation, but rather on whether otherwise "normal" people should be treated. There are also, of course, the typical warnings about adverse side effects of misusing large injections, resulting in edema, carpal tunnel syndrome, and other effects.

The Lungs

The volume and capacity of the lungs deteriorate with age, and COPD is much more common in the elderly than in younger people. According to Dr. Klatz, Dr. David Clemmons of the University of North Carolina ran a study on a group of people who had COPD with only 25% of the lung capacity and strength of normal adults.

Lung capacity is measured by how much air can be expelled after deep inhalation and rapid exhalation. The force of the exhaled air is measured in mm/Hg, or millimeters of mercury. Normal adults without COPD measure about 100 mg/Hg, and those in Dr. Clemmon's study measured only about 25 mm/Hg.

After HGH replacement therapy, the patients improved to an average of 38 mm/Hg, enough to make the patients feel significant relief. It will be interesting to see if the results improve further with continued treatment, especially since conventional medicine has very little to offer these patients.

The Cardiovascular System

Statistics tell us that heart disease, heart attacks, and stroke together are the top three causes of death in the United States. (COPD is fifth.) The good news is that research being conducted worldwide is beginning to show evidence that HGH replacement therapy can slow and even begin to reverse the effects of cardiovascular disease. But the relationship between cardiovascular disease and HGH is unusual. Too much HGH is bad, and too little is bad.

Fortunately, this U-shaped graph is very broad. At the high end, people whose pituitary produces an abnormally high amount have a disease called acromegaly, causing unusually large body size and a notably large jawbone structure. Body builders and athletes who have experimented with very large doses of HGH, like the people with acromegaly, have higher than average heart disease rates, and more heart attacks.

At the low end of the curve, people with low production of HGH, either due to disease or age, also experience high incidence of heart disease.

What are the effects of HGH replacement therapy that helps? There are several well-known observed effects on the body that also effects cardiovascular health. Dr. Bengtsson found the following beneficial effects on his patients:

- Body composition – fat mass decreases and muscle mass increases.

- Abdominal fat decreases.

- Lower LDL (bad cholesterol).

- Higher HDL (good cholesterol).

- Lower triglycerides.

- Lower fibrinogen.

- Lowered diastolic blood pressure.

- Reduced insulin resistance.

The blood pressure reduction was a surprise. Most people had thought that HGH increased blood pressure, and his research showed the exact opposite.

Atherosclerosis

Dr Bengtsson believes that future studies will show the beneficial effects of HGH therapy on atherosclerosis (hardening of the arteries). He states that this disease is actually a metabolic disorder.

Dr. Klatz explains the process in his book, previously referenced: *"While most people focus on cholesterol plaques in the artery, the real action takes place in the liver. This is the primary organ for disposing of cholesterol by transforming it into bile acids or shipping it into the gallbladder and from there to the intestines where it can be excreted from the body. Growth hormone enhances this metabolism by increasing the number of LDL receptors in the cells of the liver that remove LDL cholesterol from the circulation."*

Dr. Bengtsson states that *"This is the way to clean up the circulation from cholesterol."*

For further reading, I repeat my recommendation of Dr. Klatz's books. There he describes the research projects that are showing very exciting favorable results in other cardiovascular cases: reversing the effects of stroke and heart attacks, and reversing cardiac failure.

Body Composition

As we age, everyone notices that our bodies begin to change their shape. Pot bellies are nearly universal, and at the same time arms, legs, and shoulders get skinnier. Dr. Rudman's study at the Medical College of the University of Wisconsin reported that the bodies of young adults with pituitary disease mimicked those of his elderly patients. In six months of treatment with HGH supplementation, these patients experienced an 8.8% gain in lean body mass, a 14.4% decrease in fat mass, and skin thickened by 7.1%. This is while the untreated control group's body mass and organ size continued to decrease by 2.5 to 4.5% per year.

Obesity patients show similar results. In a double-blind, placebo controlled, crossover study, obese women lost more than 4.6 pounds of body fat, 5% reduction in total body mass, and an increase of 6 pounds of lean body mass in just five weeks.

Dr. Klatz reports that the latest results coming from Sweden show that HGH therapy is the best weapon yet against middle age weight gain and the associated problems that come along with it.

Obesity

Dr. David Clemmons, chief of endocrinology at the University of North Carolina in Chapel Hill, conducted a controlled double-blind study on obese patients. These patients were all put on the same weight-loss diets, but some were given HGH injections while others were given placebo injections. Those patients that received HGH lost weight 25% faster than those on diet alone.

This author, generally adhering to a fairly low carbohydrate diet, lost 15 pounds over the past year or two, mainly by eating less. His weight has been stable now for months. However after a few weeks on Somaderm, he experienced a flatter tummy and the loss of five additional pounds.

Body Strength

Through the presence of HGH, IGF-1 being available to cells increases their intake of amino acids (the protein building blocks), and enhances the synthesis of DNA, RNA, proteins, sugars, and carbohydrates. The result is an increase in cell size and enhanced cell division.

HGH could increase strength by increasing protein synthesis in the body's muscle cells, and also by increasing the number of muscle cells, resulting in greater strength and leaner body mass. While studies are unequivocal about leaner body mass, there is not widespread agreement about strength improvements.

In one controlled double-blind study, the significance of the increase in quadricep strength observed in those receiving HGH was deemed statistically less significant because of a small increase in strength in the control group. Increases in body strength is therefore still doubted by some, and the results of newer studies on this are coming. (This test in particular raises my suspicion about whether the results are interpreted correctly statistically. Obviously, being a double blind study, both groups had to exercise an equal amount. Not to expect or be able to account for some increase in strength in the control group sounds like a mathematics deficiency problem to me. Like Dr. Pauling had found earlier in his study of vitamin C effectiveness analyses.)

Bone Density

One of the longest reported studies on HGH replacement therapy was done in Sweden. The authors concluded that *"There are few studies that have determined the effects of long-term GH replacement on bone mineral density (BMD) in GH-deficient (GHD) adults. In this study, the effects of 10 years of GH replacement on BMD were assessed in 87 GHD adults using dual energy X-ray absorptiometry (DEXA). The results show that GH replacement induced a sustained increase in BMD at all the skeletal sites measured."*[6]

This study also serves as additional evidence of the effectiveness of low-dose daily supplementation. The doses began at less than 1 mg/day, and over the course of the study decreased to less than .5 mg/day. (A milligram of HGH is 3 IU.) Other successful studies have shown the beneficial effects of daily doses as low as .5 IU per day.

Certainly, the increase in fragility as we age is one of the greatest dangers. Many hip fractures result in hospital stays, often complicated by the contraction of disease by already immune-deficient elderly patients.

In addition to HGH supplementation, bone density can be increased by exercise, and in females, with estrogen replacement.

Skin and Hair

As we age, our skin becomes thinner and more fragile. Veins become more difficult to find for blood tests, as many elderly people painfully discover. And most visible, perhaps, are the appearance of wrinkles,

---

[6] *Ten-year GH replacement increases bone mineral density in hypopituitary patients with adult onset GH deficiency,* G Götherström, B-Å Bengtsson, I Bosæus1, G Johannsson and J Svensson, Research Centre for Endocrinology and Metabolism and Department of Clinical Nutrition, Sahlgrenska University Hospital, Gröna Stråket 8, SE-413 45 Göteborg, Sweden, 20.

which increase in number and depth as the years go by.

The effects of HGH replacement therapy on people's skin is nearly universal. Studies consistently show that skin becomes measurably thicker with continued treatment.

Research has also shown that HGH boosts collagen synthesis and improves the actual muscle mass under wrinkles. It appears that the well-researched benefit of HGH on muscle mass also appears to carry over to enhancing skin muscle tone, improving elasticity, and increasing skin thickness.

Dr. Thierry Hertoghe, at the Academy de Medicine General de Belgium from Belgium, performed a study of 48 adults, who were give a daily dose of .75 IU of prescription HGH for a two month period.

Here are the results he reported:

- Face wrinkles - 71% had fewer wrinkles

- Sagging cheeks - 75% experienced denser muscle tone

- Pouches under eyes - less visible 65%

- Skin thickness increased by 34%

- Thin lips thickened by 25%

In a renowned study by Dr. Daniel Rudman, elderly men had an increase of skin thickness an average of 7.1%. Dr. Rudman did further self-evaluation of 202 people taking HGH for six months, and the results showed that two thirds of them reported improvement in skin texture, skin thickness, and skin elasticity. In this same group, 61% observed fewer wrinkles and 38% reported new hair growth.

Dr. Chien reports *"If you give someone growth hormone you improve the collagen synthesis and increase the muscle mass underneath the wrinkles. You ae really doing medical cosmetic plastic surgery."*

A popular simple test of skin elasticity is the pinch test. Pinch the skin in the fatty area between your thumb and forefinger, and see how long it takes to flatten out. As you might expect, older people's skin takes longer.

According to Dr. Klatz, Chien frequently uses the pinch test against people he meets. He reports that when he began HGH supplementation his pinch test was typical for people in their forties. After one year, however, he began beating people in their thirties, and now even in their twenties.

Although there does not seem to be any studies yet on hair health and growth, there are many doctors who are reporting that they have patients who have sprouted new hair in balding areas, regained hair color, experienced more robust nail growth, and even more lush eye lashes. Stay tuned.

The Immune System

The effects of HGH replacement therapy on the immune system might be the least noticed but most important benefit.

The primary organ of the immune system is the thymus gland, which begins to shrink so much with age that by the age of 60 it is difficult to detect. The reason for this is unknown, but the effect of the thymus on our health is well-known.

The thymus is important in the formation of the T-cell lymphocytes, known as the foot soldiers in the fight against disease. As the thymus shrinks, the decreasing T-cells make us more vulnerable to cancer, heart disease, infectious diseases, and autoimmune disorders.

AIDS patients' loss of T-cells is what makes them vulnerable to all these diseases, which makes aging look like AIDS in slow motion.

The connection between HGH decline and the shrinking of the thymus was proven by Dr. Keith Kelly of the University of Illinois, Urbana-Champaign. He injected growth hormone into old rats, whose thymus glands had almost vanished. His exciting results were that the thymus in the old rats grew back to the size of those in the younger, robust rats.[7]

Dr. Kelley says *"Everyone considered that the thymus went away and you couldn't get it back. But clearly that was incorrect. It was not due to a genetic defect. It was not programmed to go away in the sense that you couldn't get it*

---

[7] G.H. Kelley, *GH3 Pituitary Adenoma Implants Can Reverse Thymic Aging*, Proceedings of the National Academy of Sciences.

back. You could get it back by using a treatment. And that treatment is growth hormone. The synthesis of interleukin 2 by T-cells in old rats goes down. If you give them growth hormone, it comes back up."

Israeli scientists have confirmed Dr. Kelley's results also in dogs and mice. Dr. Klatz lists the immune activities that growth hormone improves:

- Manufacture of new antibodies.

- Increased production of T-cells and interleukin 2.

- More activity in disease-fighting white blood cells.

- More active NK cells that protect against cancer.

- More bacteria-engulfing macrophages.

- Increased production of new red blood cells.

- Increased production of white blood cells that fight microorganisms.

David Kahnsari and Thomas Gustad at the North Dakota State University in Fargo showed that, sure enough, improved immune systems increases life span, as might be expected. They carried out an experiment that showed that mice treated with growth hormone lived 33% longer lives than expected.

Wasting

Elderly people often lose interest in food, causing them to "waste away." Many elderly hospital patients and probably more than half of nursing home resident are malnourished.

Dr. Fran Kaiser, M.D., conducted a double-blind study of ten malnourished elderly men who were consistently losing weight by not eating enough. Five of the men were given growth hormone, and five a placebo treatment. All the men were excreting nitrogen, which is a sign of muscle wasting.

After six weeks, those receiving HGH had increased appetites, lower nitrogen excretion, and gained weight. The other group, on placebo, continued the wasting, and refused to eat more in spite of the staff encouraging them to do so.[8]

It shouldn't be a surprise that the five treated with HGH also showed improved optimism and rosy outlooks that accompanied their increased appetite and feeling of well-being.

Sexual Function

One of the most disappointing signs of aging is the decline of sexual function in both men and women. Women experience menopause, and men experience andropause. Andropause is not as sudden or noticeable as menopause, but it happens nonetheless.

As we age, our sex organs, along with most of our other organs, begin shrinking in size. Their function is also impaired, and sexual pleasure and activity fall dramatically.

There is no doubt that there are psychological causes in addition to the physical causes, and one may cause the other (in either direction --you choose). But the physical effects can be measured, and are nearly universal in both men and women.

Dr. Klatz's books devote much more space to the subject than is possible here, but the positive effects of HGH supplementation seem to be helpful in both physical and psychological ways. Who wouldn't be happier reliving their 20's and 30's again?

Is there a connection between the decline in HGH as we age and the decline in sexual function? According to Dr. Klatz, Drs. Chien and Terry did the first analysis of that in a study comprised of 202 people (172 men). After HGH replacement therapy, 75% reported increases in sexual performance or frequency. 62% reported longer, more sustained erections.

As Dr. Klatz points out, it is always possible that the placebo effect is responsible. But researchers also know that placebo effects are not long-lasting, and the reported effects from HGH have been noticed for months and years.

Some changes are enhanced by previously-discussed benefits of HGH: improved circulation, lower LDL and higher HDL, boosted production of testosterone and estrogen, improved body shape and diminished fat content, and improved outlook and feelings of quality

---

[8] Fran Kaiser, associate director of geriatrics at the Geriatric Research, Education, and Clinical Center of the Veterans Administration in St. Louis.

of life.

Specifically, the changes are noticed in a number of areas:

- Organ size, in which the penis and clitoris stop shrinking and begin to return to their original size.

- Re-hydration of the vagina, which makes sex more pleasant.

- Stronger and longer-lasting erections.

- Increased libido for both sexes.

- Enhanced orgasms for both sexes.

Many of the testimonials are from doctors who began treating themselves after witnessing the effects of HGH on their patients. More than one doctor insists that both parties in a marriage be treated or the marriage may wind up in trouble!

Changes in libido and sexual performance and pleasure are most noticeable in older patients, many of whom began HGH replacement therapy for other reasons. Patients in their 60's, 70's, and 80's report the fun and excitement of feeling and acting like they did decades earlier.

Being an experienced researcher, this author is convinced that the proper use of HGH can slow, and in some cases, reverse some of the symptoms of aging. However the cost (usually about $1,500 per month) and the inconvenience (two injections per day) discourage most people from taking advantage of HGH replacement therapy.

Now, however, things have changed dramatically. Today there is an affordable (about $150 per month) and simple (applying gel to the skin) method of performing HGH replacement therapy at home, by yourself.

HGH Gel

4 Somaderm

Somaderm[TM] is the trade name of the HGH Gel that is the primary subject of this book. Its story actually goes back more than a dozen years, when it was a popular but little-recognized homeopathic transdermal gel invented and manufactured by a company in Northern California.

Alex Goldstein had to take over the family health supplement business while still in college, but wound up running it, growing it, and, as his education and experience increased, adding more and more of his own products to the mix.

His remarkable story does not need to be repeated here, but is available on the company website, www.newulife.com. The primary reason Somaderm is one of the products that attracted the most attention was the extremely high reorder rate among its users, along with their enthusiastic testimonials.

Furthermore, it answered the need for an affordable and convenient way for people to take advantage of low-dose, high-frequency supplementation of the human growth hormone somatropin. Avoiding twice-daily injections and at a small fraction of the cost of traditional LDHF treatment, his homeopathic formula had an additional advantage of providing a number of substances that boost people's own glandular system to increase its own production of HGH and other important anti-aging hormones.

After receiving its FDA listing, investors (reportedly including one or more Shark Tank stars) began contacting Alex. The opportunity to start a bigger business based primarily on Somaderm was a very attractive opportunity.

The Business Model

There are not very many ways to get a new product to a mass market unless it is just a new product from a large well-established business.

Mass markets typically require the company to produce huge amounts of inventory, and to spread that inventory among distributors whose primary efforts are to coax retailers into giving space on their shelves or on their counters to a new product, usually replacing an existing product. There is probably another layer of wholesalers in between the company and the retailers. This is an extremely expensive and risky way to introduce a product that does not already come from a large recognized company. It requires outside investors to invest large amounts of money, in exchange for ownership, of course. And where does the inventor wind up? Who knows? Certainly not running his own business any more.

Another way to reach the market is on the Internet. Build a website, do a good job of SEO (Search Engine Optimization), and hope Google helps find you customers. That's certainly an affordable solution, and preferable to the first one described above. But it is slow and unsure, and there is not a lot company management can do to accelerate it. And it is slow to show the most important effects of a marketing program: word of mouth.

In any method of distribution and sales, there is no more effective way to accelerate a product's acceptance and sales as word of mouth. People telling their friends that they like something has more effect on the friends' decision to purchase than anything else.

So why not use a form of distribution that relies mainly on word of mouth advertising? Multi-level marketing (MLM) is often chosen as the best alternative. It does not require nearly as great an initial investment, it does not require convincing retailers to give up some shelf space, it does not require filling warehouses full of unsold inventory, and it leaves the founder in the driver's seat overseeing his own company's growth.

MLM takes what would otherwise be the money spent on wholesalers, distributors, and sales agents and puts it directly in the pockets of those people who are spreading the word using personal introductions and recommendations to the sales prospects. The financial rewards are going where it is earned. It is an extremely fair system, rewarding regular people for their efforts and contributions.

That is the business model for the distribution and sale of Somaderm. The details are described on the company's web site, as noted previously.

The Product

Somaderm is made up of 21 ingredients, three of which are listed as the active ingredients.

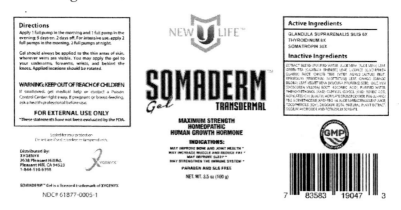

Figure 6.   The Somaderm Gel Label

Glandula Suprarenalis Suis, 6X

The first listed ingredient, glandula suprarenalis suis, means adrenal gland extract. The adrenal gland is responsible for may cellular functions, and adrenal fatigue is accompanied by the following symptoms:[9]

- Fatigue

- Body aches

---

[9] https://www.mayoclinic.org/diseases-conditions/addisons-disease/expert-answers/adrenal-fatigue/faq-20057906

- Unexplained weight loss

- Low blood pressure

- Lightheadedness

- Loss of body hair

- Skin discoloration (hyperpigmentation)

Adrenal fatigue is a term applied to a collection of nonspecific symptoms, such as body aches, fatigue, nervousness, sleep disturbances, and digestive problems.

Like aging in general, most physicians (Mayo Clinic included) do not recognize adrenal fatigue as a disease, and don't agree how it should be treated. But the symptoms for many people are real, and increase as they age. The adrenals, along with most of your other glands, shrink as you age, and their effectiveness declines.

Adrenal insufficiency can be detected by blood tests, and can be shown to be worsened by physical or mental stress.

So like HGH replacement therapy, returning the adrenal gland effectiveness to the point where it had been earlier in life, and usually before symptoms appear, is a perfectly acceptable to many doctors and researchers who believe that, disease or not, aging can and should be treated.

Thyroidinum (Bovine) 8X

This is a thyroid extract intended to offset the decrease in the output from your own thyroid as you grow older.

At first, you may barely notice the symptoms of hypothyroidism, such as fatigue and weight gain, or you may simply attribute them to getting older. But as your metabolism continues to slow, you may develop more-obvious signs and symptoms. Hypothyroidism signs and symptoms may include:[10]

- Fatigue

- Increased sensitivity to cold

---

[10] https://www.mayoclinic.org/diseases-conditions/hypothyroidism/symptoms-causes/syc-20350284

- Constipation
- Dry skin
- Weight gain
- Puffy face
- Hoarseness
- Muscle weakness
- Elevated blood cholesterol level
- Muscle aches, tenderness and stiffness
- Pain, stiffness or swelling in your joints
- Heavier than normal or irregular menstrual periods
- Thinning hair
- Slowed heart rate
- Depression
- Impaired memory

Because most of us experience one or more of these symptoms as we age, it is very appropriate that this hormone extract be included in Somaderm.

Many doctors fear that hypothyroidism may be on the rise due to a general lack of iodine in our bodies. Many years ago, scientists discovered that this disorder could be avoided by iodizing table salt, which virtually wiped out the incidence of goiter, for example. But recently, salt gets a bad rap for supposedly causing high blood pressure, and many who don't avoid salt are instead using sea salt, which contains virtually no iodine.

The inclusion of thyroid extract in Somaderm makes a good deal of sense, since it is one more weapon against the decrease in crucial hormones that decrease as we age.

Somatropin 30X

Somatropin, of course, is the hormone that has been the main subject of this book. Its source, use, and results have been documented here and in many other publications.

Of course, that doesn't mean that its use is not controversial. There is general agreement that in low-dose high-frequency applications that there are no side effects. And there is also general agreement as to the conditions it improves in those with impaired pituitary function. The disagreement in medical circles is whether aging is a condition that should be treated. My vote is Yes.

There are those that complain that the amounts of these ingredients, particularly HGH (somatropin) are too small to be effective. Here is where people need to understand and subscribe to (or not) with homeopathic medicine.

What do 6X, 8X, and 30X Mean?

These are designations from the world of homeopathic medicine. These terms, and variations of them, are used worldwide to designate the strength or dilution of the named ingredient.

Homeopathic medicine practitioners and followers do not believe that the absolute strength of an ingredient is the only factor in its effectiveness. They believe that the preparation method is very important in supplying the resulting formula with the potency it needs to be effective in treating the patient.

The classic preparation method for preparing homeopathic compounds is one of successive dilutions and processing, usually involving fairly violent mixing processes, such as shaking.

For example, a 3X ingredient may be processed by adding one ounce of the undiluted ingredient to 10 ounces of solvent; usually water, ethyl alcohol, or a mixture of both. This is shaken vigorously, and then one ounce of that is added to another 10 ounces of solvent, and again mixed. A third time (3X) of adding one ounce of that to another 10 ounces of solvent results in the final 3X ingredient that is used either by itself or in combination with other ingredients. Thus the final 3X mixture contains one part in one thousand of the original ingredient.

The three is essentially an exponent of 10 describing the strength of the final mixture. The larger the number the weaker the solution. In Somaderm, as is always the case, the ingredients are listed in the order of decreasing quantity, which is 3, then 6, and then 30.

You math people will realize that 30X is very small, which is not of concern to homeopathic doctors. If, however, you are a homeopathic skeptic, you may want to boost your HGH intake by adding additional supplementation, as I do, with a 6X somatropin product for about $15 per month.

Very few people interested in wellness and age extension take only one product anyway. Somatropin, as do even most multivitamins, contains vitamin C, for example, but not in the quantities I use in my daily regimen. (I wonder sometimes how old you have to get before people start asking you for nutritional advice instead of giving it.)

The Other Ingredients

The remaining ingredients are all known wellness supplements to one degree or another. This book is not intended to cover such a wide field, but all of these ingredients either support your well-being, or boost your natural hormonal secretions, or are replacing nutrients that are not adequately available to our bodies either because of age, lifestyle, eating habits, or disease.

Expectations

As with anything new you try, it is important to manage your expectations. As I stated early in this book, somatropin has an effect on every cell in your body, but not all the cellular effects are fast enough to be noticed initially.

For example, improvements in brain function can be noticed sooner than an improvement in skin tone, even though your skin cells may begin to react almost immediately.

The official Somaderm list of expectations follows very nearly the same order as we discussed earlier in the book from the results of dozens of carefully monitored and documented tests. It is important that these expectations, because everyone is different and Somaderm is not a medicine, be viewed as possible outcomes of treatment, and have not been certified or verified by the FDA or any other agency.

General Expected Benefits

1st Month

- May experience improved stamina*
- May experience increased energy*
- May experience deeper sleep*
- May experience vivid dreams*

2nd Month

- May experience muscle definition*
- May experience heightened libido*
- May experience healthier skin*
- May experience increased strength*
- May experience weight loss*
- May experience improved vision*

3rdMonth

Benefits from Months 1 and 2 are heightened.*

- May experience enhanced focus*
- May experience hair growth*
- May experience enhanced muscle mass*
- May experience PMS symptoms reduced*
- May experience greater flexibility*
- May experience healthier nails*
- May experience improved joint mobility*
- May experience increase in sexual desire*
- May experience alleviation in some menopausal symptoms*

4th Month

Benefits from months 1, 2 & 3 are not only heightened, but also more consistent*

Please understand that although results may seem to vanish, your body may be utilizing the HGH hormone for tissue repair. Tests indicate that the benefits resume with continued use.*

5*th* Month

• May experience significant weight loss*

• May experience greater improvements in skin texture & appearance*

• May experience skin has greater elasticity*

• May experience reduction of the appearance of wrinkles*

• May experience hair becomes even healthier & thicker*

6*th* Month

Benefits from previous months are heightened even more.*

• May experience cellulite greatly diminishes*

• May experience improved immune system*

• May experience pain and general soreness diminishes*

• May experience wounds heal quicker*

• May experience greater metabolic output*

• May experience grayed hair begins to return to natural color*

• May experience reduction in LDL cholesterol*

• May experience blood pressure normalizes*

• May experience heart rate improves*

*These benefits are based on the experiences of customers using Somaderm Gel over the past 13 years.

Mentioned earlier were three tests to monitor how you are improving: The Pinch Test, Concentration, and the Falling Ruler tests.

Test Yourself

I recommend that you prove to yourself that your improvements are real and not imaginary by performing these tests in the beginning of your Somaderm journey, and monthly thereafter. The results of these tests are objective, and can be measured.

The Pinch Test

This is a skin elasticity test. Pinch the skin in the fatty area between your thumb and forefinger, and note the time it takes to flatten out. See if this test performed monthly shows an increase in your skin thickness and elasticity as the flattening time decreases.

Concentration

Concentration is a kid's card game, and if you are over 50 I'll bet a kid will beat you every time – at least until your HGH levels get back up. The game consists of laying all 52 cards face down on the table, and the players take turns turning two cards over at a time. If the cards match, the player keeps them, but otherwise puts them back where they came from. Now remember where those cards are, because when later you turn over a card, you will be allowed to keep it if you can remember where a matching card is. Whoever has the most cards at the end wins.

Play this game when you start using Somaderm, and repeat monthly thereafter against the same person (who is not taking it.) I predict that you will be pleasantly surprised at your memory improvement.

The Falling Ruler

Catching the falling ruler is an excellent and easy test for your reflexes. Have a friend hold a yardstick vertically in front of you, and place your thumb and index finger about an inch apart at the 18 inch mark. Then have your friend drop the ruler unexpectedly, and you catch it as fast as you can. (If you're *really* slow, start at the 20 or 36 inch mark!) Make a note of the inch mark where your fingers land, and keep track of your progress monthly as you continue using your Somaderm.

• Managing Expectations

It is important to not only manage your own expectations, but those to whom you introduce Somaderm (or any other supplement). I read a review of a health product recently from someone who gave the product one star and complained that he had used it for two weeks and hadn't seen results. Not only has he cheated himself out of possible health improvements, he may have discouraged others from trying.

5 Additional Age-Fighting Supplements

I have studied nutrition for many decades. I'm not a nutritionist, I'm an electrical engineer and physicist. Most of my achievements have been the result of exhaustive research, so I know how to do it. You have to learn to research the sources as much as the subject.

We used to go to libraries and painfully go through the stacks, checking out as many books as we could carry, and then hoping that what we needed to know was inside. What we would have given for a search engine!

Now, with the Internet, you can get 50 million results from your search in milliseconds. However, the Internet is not fact-checked by anyone, so it is up to you to decide who to believe. This is often not easy, even if the source is a reliable institution. Sometimes, even good news looks like bad news (or no news) if the facts are interpreted poorly. Dr. Pauling's work is an outstanding example of this.

Vitamin C

When a group of engineers and physicists that worked for me read, as I did, *Vitamin C and the Common Cold*, by Dr. Linus Pauling, we paid attention. Linus Pauling, one of the few scientists in the world who had won two Nobel Prizes, surprised us and many others by not conducting any original research, but by analyzing the results of other earlier studies.

He found that the researchers misinterpreted the results of their own studies due to poor math skills. He discovered volumes of work denigrating the importance of vitamin C supplementation that were exactly wrong. And every doctor who turns up their nose at "expensive urine" are still living in the past -- about four decades ago.

(I always point out that just because some vitamins appear in urine doesn't mean that your body does not need them. Water is also in your urine...)

Back then, we couldn't find a source for crystalline vitamin C anywhere but our local industrial chemical company, so I purchased it there and made it a fringe benefit in the coffee room. At the time, ascorbic acid (vitamin C) was mostly used for agricultural applications, it being a powerful anti-bacterial and anti-fungal agent. It is also used commercially as a powerful anti-oxidant, which keeps your commercial applesauce and guacamole from turning brown on the shelf.

The modest investment in making C available free to employees paid off many times over as the hours of sick leave shrank over the coming months.

One lesson learned just regarding vitamin C: the British Navy discovered long ago that limes prevented scurvy and began a campaign that ruled the world's oceans because the competing navies' sailors were all sick with scurvy, but it was another 100 years before it was discovered that it was vitamin C that did the trick. The symptoms of scurvy are similar to those you would expect from accelerated aging, which led Dr. Pauling to call our "normal" state of health "sub-clinical scurvy."

Chromium

We read *The Trace Minerals and Man*, by Henry A. Schroeder, M.D. and were impressed by his research on lab mice, and how he could cause and then reverse various disorders by adding or subtracting elements from their diets. There came some more changes in our habits and diets. Schroeder tied each discovery to the real world; if chromium was shown to decrease the incidence of arteriosclerosis, then how did that connect with natural sources and incidence of disease?

Chromium was so important in such a wide variety of health problems that we sought a dietary supplement for it, and there were none. We assigned one of the mechanical engineers the problem (he had one more chemistry course than the rest of us). He never came up with anything we could stand, but within a few months chromium picolinate was suddenly made available, which is now practically a universal multivitamin ingredient.

Co-enzyme Q$_{10}$

CoQ$_{10}$ is especially important for heart health, and should be part of your regimen. This is especially true if you are on cholesterol-lowering medicine, which counteracts it.

If you read a book about it, you will notice that one of the first effects that it has on your body is the promotion of dental health. It fights and prevents gum disease, and people who take it regularly don't have periodontal disease. Because it also promotes heart health, the same people have lower rates of heart disease.

Just like clockwork, every few years there are a bunch of news articles linking heart disease and periodontal disease, and they can't find the link. They keep trying to find a bacteria or something that makes gum disease cause heart problems, or vice versa. It makes one realize how low the quality of health reporting is in the common media. Unfortunately, I have talked to many medical doctors who also don't understand the link between heart disease and gum disease.

Most people use a variety of vitamins and other supplements, and it isn't necessary or possible to list them here. Generally, we all gradually develop our own routines depending upon what we and our doctors deem suitable and beneficial. You should do the same.

All our nutritional work, which was fun and fascinating, was done on our lunch hours. We had to keep concentrating on our main mission: developing and producing the photon-counting detectors I helped invent and produce for both spectrographs on the Hubble Space Telescope.

Melatonin and DHEA

Dr. Klatz, in his books, also looks carefully at research being done by others, and goes into greater detail than I possibly could in this book. As do many anti-aging researchers and doctors, he recommends melatonin, DHEA, and a variety of amino acids and vitamins to help the body in many ways, including helping your body produce what HGH it can. Again, I encourage those of you who want to get into the details to buy his books, as referenced previously.
'

It is generally thought that people with cancer should not use DHEA until more evidence is available.

In general, please consult your physician about any nutritional regimen you choose to use.

Here's to Youthful Health and Happiness!

About the Author

Mr. Choisser received his degree in electrical engineering at the University of Arizona, and took graduate courses in mathematics at Syracuse University. He is an Air Force veteran, having been an officer in the Data Processing Branch of the Intelligence and Electronic Warfare Directorate of Rome Air Development Center, Griffiss AFB, New York. He and his officemates were some of 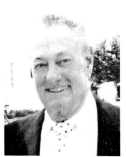 the earliest pioneers in the field of Artificial Intelligence. Upon leaving the service, he was awarded the Air Force Systems Command Award for Scientific Achievement.

In his business career, his first career involved the development of low-light-level sensors for military and scientific uses. He is one of the co-inventors and developer of the Digicon, the multi-channel photon counting image tubes used in both of the original Hubble Space Telescope spectrographs. He was awarded special recognition for this work by the NASA Goddard Space Flight Center.

His longest career was designing and building industrial versions of the IBM PC. His work with industry and the military resulted in the use of Microsoft DOS and Windows in a wide variety of non-desktop applications. He was a speaker and sponsor of many technical conferences and was editor-in-chief of the Windows CE Tech Journal, a Miller-Freeman publication.

His hobbies have always been nutritional studies, airplanes, gardening, cooking, and golf.

He is also the founder of Readerplace Books, LLC. The mission of Readerplace is to provide authors an affordable alternative to the conventional publishing industry for their eBooks and print books. Visit www.readerplace.com for more information.

John's recipes and cooking tips are found at www.cookingdude.com. His Somaderm™ web site is at www.hghgelcream.com.